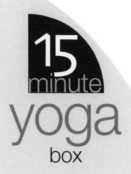

15 minute

yoga
box

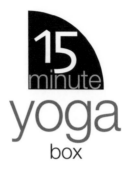

15 minute yoga box

Discover serenity, focus, and health in
just 15 minutes a day

Barbara Currie

**BARNES
& NOBLE**

NEW YORK

Text © Barbara Currie 2003
© HarperColllins*Publishers* 2003

Previously published as *10-Minute Yoga Workouts* and *Look 15 Years Younger:
The 15-Minute-a-Day Yoga Plan*

This 2003 edition published by Barnes & Noble, Inc.
by arrangement with *HarperThorsons*, an imprint of HarperCollins*Publishers*

Photography by Guy Hearn

ISBN-13 978-0-7607-4707-0
ISBN-10 0-7607-4707-5

Printed and bound in China

10 9 8 7 6 5 4 3 2 1

Not all exercises are suitable for everyone. To reduce the risk to you, please
consult your doctor before beginning this exercise program. The instructions
andadvicepresented are in no way intended as a substitute for medical
guidance. The writer and publishers of this book do not accept any
responsibility for any injury or accident as a result of following this
exercise program.

Contents

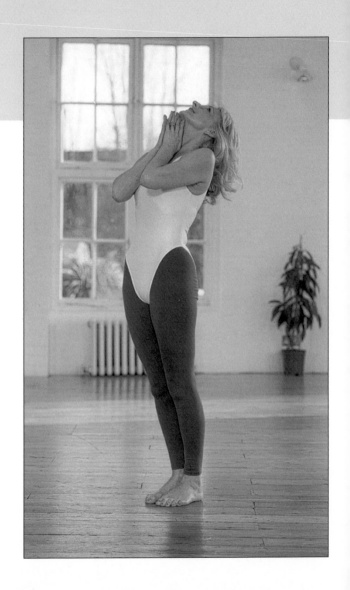

Introduction

"Whatever you can do or dream you can begin it. Boldness has genius, magic, and power in it. Begin it now."

Goethe

I have been learning yoga for many years and from time to time I received some jolts or wake-up calls as ancient legends and parables were recited to us, teaching us age-old truths. This is one of my favorites. It goes something like this:

"Once upon a time there was a king with the most amazing palaces, beautiful gardens and parks, servants to cater for his every need, and riches beyond his wildest dreams. He did not, however, enjoy good health or happiness. He desired these two qualities more than anything else in life and sent his servants out far and wide to find someone with the secret that they could share with him. Eventually after many, many years of combing his kingdom they found an old lady in the mountains who made a very special herbal brew. The King sent for her immediately but she refused to come saying that the brew had to be made freshly and the herbs only grew around her small house in the mountains. So one day the King, reluctantly, went to see the old lady. She insisted that he stayed in her house alone with her for at least a week and again, reluctantly, the King agreed. The old lady gave him simple, fresh food and took him for long walks in the beautiful mountains that surrounded her home. They watched the sunrise and sunset and marvelled at the bright starry skies. Each night before bed she dosed him with the special herbal mix saying it would bring him health and happiness. He slept better than he had done in years. At the end of the week he said happily the herbal brew had worked wonders and he needed to take a large supply back with him to his palace for which he would reward her handsomely. The old lady replied, "There was nothing in the brew that had any special power at all. The secret of happiness and health is and has always been within ourselves."

All she had done was reveal this to him.

Isn't this what we are really looking for? When you are happy and healthy inside, your face and body glows with a youthful inner radiance that no amount of expensive face cream or cosmetic surgery can give you. The yogis of ancient India realized this well over 5000 years ago.

Yoga can literally change your life: it's an enjoyable route to a firmer body, greater flexibility, and improved energy levels too. In just

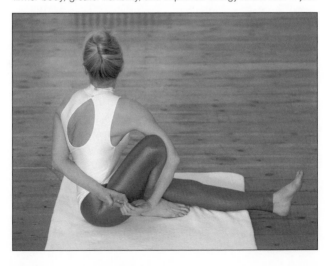

15 minutes every day you can reap the benefits of this age-old system. *15-Minute Yoga Box* adapts this brilliant 5000-year-old practice to the needs and lifestyles of people living in the twenty-first century. Having studied and taught yoga for nearly 30 years, I have spent a lot of time listening to my pupils and realize that only a lucky few have time to do an hour's yoga a day. This is why we have put together three 15-minute card sequences for everyone to work on, young and old, beginners and old hands. Everyone can work through the three sequences at their own pace. Beginners will perhaps find themselves holding poses for the minimum amount of time recommended, while those of you who are more advanced can take the poses to a deeper level. The important thing to remember about yoga is that it is not competitive – no one should force themselves into a position where they are not comfortable. Gradual change is the key to yoga!

Each of the sequences mixes the different aspects of yoga: breathing, balances, floorwork, standing poses, stretches. Relaxation is the end point of any yoga practice and so each of the 15-minute sequences ends with a relaxation exercise.

I would like you to start every day with one of these sequences. They will keep your spine and joints really strong and flexible while toning virtually every muscle in your body. They are a wonderful energizing start for every day – 15 minutes that will give you a perfect balanced workout for mind and body, changing both your body and your life. It's only 15 minutes every day but you'll be amazed how quickly those 15 minutes add up into noticeable benefits, in the clarity of your mind and the tone of your body.

Using 15-Minute Yoga Box

Yoga is not only about your body and exercise – it also has tremendous effects on the mind, helping focus and aiding concentration. So as well as the sequences on the cards we also look in this book at aspects of yoga beyond the postures.

First of all, in Chapter 1 I look at the principles, philosophy, and theory of yoga, this amazing system for helping you to live life to the fullest extent. The history of yoga is the subject of Chapter 2 – and it's an amazing history of an age-old practice that is still so relevant to our lives now. Meditation and visualization, two of yoga's

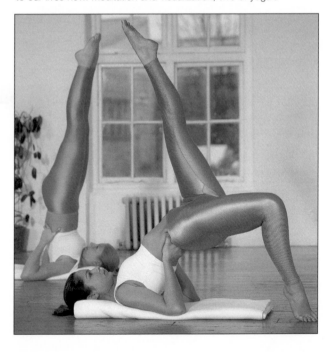

essential foundations and two of your most important tools to use for healthier, happier lives are the subject of Chapter 3. Chapter 4 takes us into the practice of yoga itself, and the practicalities of how to begin on your own journey into the world of yoga.

In Chapter 5 we move beyond the exercises and practice of yoga to take a look at the complete health picture – yoga is after all a holistic practice, meaning that it involves the whole person. I discuss the importance of meditation and how you can use this powerful tool to help keep you relaxed, calm, and focused. Diet is another essential component of yoga, and you will learn about the importance of selecting foods that will build your health and vitality. There is a chance to try my own personal diet plan, which has helped literally thousands of people to their best shape ever. Although yoga works on a holistic level, some people are particularly keen to know how yoga can help with specific health problems, and so I have included in Chapter 5 some information about common health issues.

First Principles: the Philosophy of Yoga

> "To the dull mind all nature is leaden. To the illuminated
> mind the whole world burns and sparkles with light."
>
> Ralph Waldo Emerson

The word "yoga" means union of body, mind, and spirit with the universal spirit. The yogis of ancient India realized that for perfect health and inner peace, both body and mind must work together in perfect harmony. Yoga's combination of intricate physical postures, deep breathing exercises, balances, relaxation, and meditation combine into the perfect discipline to relieve stress, calm the mind, and tone the entire body, both inside and out.

In his quest to earn more, do more, and have more, modern man subjects himself to increased physical and mental stress. The pace of life is now so fast that few of us have time to enjoy the present moment and just be. Continued stress on both body and mind increases our vulnerability to disease.

Unfortunately, although medicine has made many amazing breakthroughs in the West over the last 100 years, the focus continues to be on treating diseases and not their causes. This is where yoga can help us all so much. Stress or tension literally strangles our bodies, inhibiting blood flow to our tissues. Yoga's beautiful physical movements, combined with deep breathing exercises, will carefully rid the body of tension and stimulate the movement of oxygen-rich blood to our cells, so providing them with the nutrients that they require. As well as toning all our muscles, the physical exercises will also strengthen our bones and keep our spine and joints flexible. The lymphatic system, which fights infection and carries away toxins, is inhibited during times of stress, but as yoga carefully smoothes away the tension, it can resume its natural functions.

Serene Living

Yoga's calming balances necessitate tremendous concentration and so they take the mind off its day-to-day activities, giving it a rest. The most difficult thing to discipline, however, is the human mind. Here again yoga offers us many techniques, from breathing exercises to relaxation and meditation, which may be used to calm a turbulent mind. Gradually, and with continued practice, the combined discipline of the exercises, together with the breathing and meditation, will help us to achieve the peace and calm we desire. And just as stress inhibits our energy flow, a calm and peaceful mind will lead to abundant energy and that genuine "good-to-be-alive" feeling.

Eventually, we stop looking elsewhere for our pleasures and concentrate on "looking within", disciplining our mind to search inside ourselves for our joy and happiness. We then start to enjoy the present moment, and listen to our gut instincts, finally achieving self-realization and finding the true health and happiness that is within us all.

What is Yoga?

Realizing that for positive health, happiness, and peace of mind the body and mind must work together, the yogis developed this

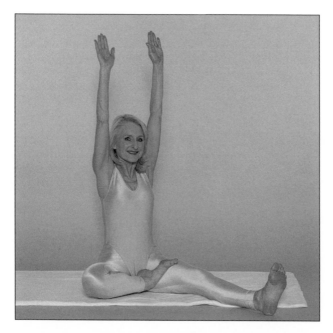

wonderful system of personal development – the science of yoga. Yoga is comprised of slow, deep, healthy breathing practices to stimulate oxygen to every cell, physical exercises to tone 100% of the body both inside and out; balancing postures to strengthen the body and help us learn the power of concentration and focus; inverted positions to reverse the adverse aging effects of gravity; stretching movements to keep the joints and spine in perfect condition; deep relaxation to help us release tension and relax; and meditation for calm deep inner peace.

The exercises coupled with a healthy diet keep the body in radiant health, the body becomes firm and beautiful, the skin glows with health, posture is corrected, stresses and strains vanish, and agility and tremendous flexibility is maintained. In my opinion yoga is the best elixir of youth and by practicing daily you will soon start to reap its magical benefits.

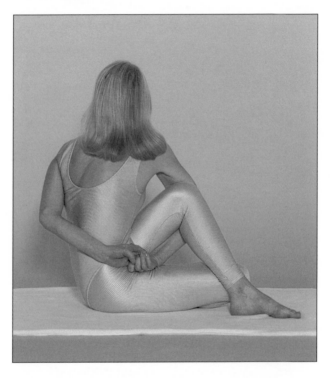

Inside each and every one of us is a force of energy called "prana", literally translated as "life force." This life-force flows freely through the body in youth but can dwindle with age if the body isn't cared for correctly, resulting in such things as lack of energy, stiffness in joints, tension, insomnia, obesity, depression, and senility together with poor posture, wrinkled, sagging skin, and dull, thin hair.

With yoga we come to realize that it is possible to stimulate the vital force within us. This doesn't come about by applying a miracle cream to our face or by sweating it out in the gym, but by proper breathing, stretching, and working our bodies so that tensions blocking the life-force around every organ, gland, nerve, tendon, cell, blood vessel, joint, and bone are released and the body becomes nourished, revitalized, and perfectly toned from WITHIN ITSELF. This, combined with alleviating stress, deep relaxation and meditation, and programming the mind to THINK and BE strong, energetic, and youthful, is the real secret to a fulfilled life.

The Seven Essential Secrets of Yoga

1 The Secret of Energy

The body has a natural energy flow which gives rise to a wonderful feeling of glowing health and wellbeing. It is, however, easily blocked or interrupted by feelings of tension, worry, anger, guilt, depression, etc.

The tensions of the mind lead to tension in the body, which can weaken the body and can eventually lead to disease. Yoga gets rid of tension by stretching the entire body from top to toe, both inside and outside. This is coupled with yoga's deep breathing which increases the oxygen level in the bloodstream. By stretching out tension, breathing deeply, and then performing postures with your head below your heart, oxygen is carefully stimulated to reach all the body's parts including the brain and as a result you will feel and look refreshed and revitalized on finishing your yoga workout.

As you continue your yoga practice on a daily basis you will find your whole body starts to feel better. You will start to understand that daily stretching to unblock your energy zones, eating fresh, vital foods, learning to relax, and meditating to calm your mind and receive new ideas puts new life into you. Your energy levels are restored and you acquire a new and real zest for life.

An extra benefit comes from visualizing energy flowing through your entire system as you perform your yoga postures and, as you concentrate on doing the movements, all negative thoughts will slip from your mind. These are the main drainers of your energy, no matter how tired you are before you start your yoga you will feel calm, focused, and energized afterwards.

2 The Secret of Perfect Shape

Yoga works 100% of the body, carefully stretching, toning, and firming all the muscles in accordance with their natural movements. This gives the body a beautiful shape, corrects posture, rebalances weak areas, corrects ugly, fatty deposits, and gives the body the famous streamlined yoga look. Yoga will never give you a bulky, tight, muscular appearance as this is totally against yoga principles. If you tighten your muscles you are like a puppet whose strings have been tightened, inhibiting the natural flexibility of the body and so limiting its movement. This leads to unnatural aging and stiffness.

Firmness of the muscles is essential to prevent the skin sagging and wrinkling and also to keep the internal organs in their correct place. Nothing looks worse than a dropped abdomen and movements such as the Abdominal Lift are brilliant for keeping this

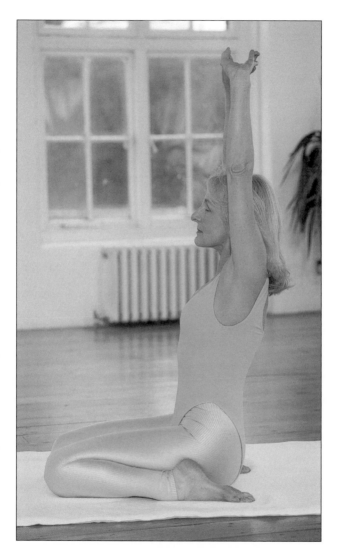

area firm, toned, and youthful. The bottom is toned and the back strengthened with movements like the Full Locust (see card 28). The thighs get an amazing workout with the balances and the Warrior Postures (see cards 23 and 24). The arms are perfectly toned with Chest Expansion (see card 22), Pose of a Mountain (see card 21), and Cow (see card 29). The face and neck area become very youthful with the head and neck exercises, and the hair regains its luster by stimulating the scalp, and finally the aging effects of gravity are carefully reversed by yoga's inverted postures which do wonders for the way we look and feel.

> **"Grace, beauty, strength, energy and firmness adorn the body through yoga."**
> Yoga sutra 111.4.7

3 The Secret of Concentration and Focus

Once you start yoga you realize that it is much more than an exercise system. The movements are quite intricate and this necessitates that you give full attention to what you are doing. By concentrating on the movement you are totally involved in the present moment and your mind is given relief from your normal day-to-day activities, so helping it to clear and giving it a rest. This means that after the yoga class your mind is calmer and much more able to deal with everyday problems, and your workload will seem easier. The balances of yoga necessitate total concentration and by focusing on a spot to help us balance physically we calm, clear, and balance the mind.

You see, feel, and take in a huge amount of stimuli from your environment. Your mind cannot possibly take in all this so it filters out all but a small amount. Your personal selection is very individual and controlled solely by your way of interpreting the things around you. If we continually focus on something and keep it in our mind it will grow stronger, whereas if we take our focus away it will gradually wither and disappear.

> **"We do not see things as they are, we see them as we are."**
> The Talmud

How does this relate to our bodies? Enormously. Every day focus on excellent health, beautiful body shape, your body radiant with energy, and your life filled with exciting new ideas and projects. See yourself as happy, beautiful, young, and vital. As you step into your shower imagine you are stepping into the fountain of youth, which will renew and refresh you daily. Do this daily for a week and feel the difference.

4 The Secret of Flexibility

When you meet someone for the very first time don't you notice

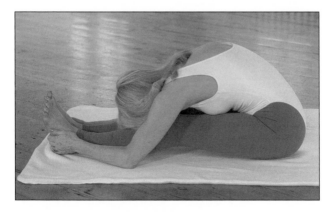

their stance and posture? Don't you notice their vitality if they stand or sit up straight and move with a relaxed agility? However, on the other hand, if the person walks and sits stiffly don't they immediately look uncomfortable?

Yoga again realized that for lifelong flexibility in both spine and joints it is necessary to work the joints carefully and in all possible directions of movement. By doing this we stimulate the flow of synovial fluid over the shiny cartilage covering of the bone surfaces of the joints. This acts as joint oil to ensure that the joint moves smoothly and also gives nourishment to the cartilage. Correct exercise also strengthens the muscles around the joint giving it support. Yoga will also add to the elasticity of your ligaments and tendons and can help to remove the calcium deposits that can collect around the joint surface so helping to keep your joints flexible for life.

A major yoga teaching is "you are as young as your spine is flexible." This is so true – just watch people and you will find that delightful ageless quality in people with a flexible spine. The spine has six directions of movement: forwards, backwards, side to side, and twisting in both directions. However, in our normal waking state over 90% of our time is spent bending forwards, without correction this can easily lead to the dreaded stoop. For perfect spinal health and flexibility the spine needs exercising daily all six ways, and the three miracle sequences will help you achieve this.

5 The Secret of Perfect Weight

In yoga we don't huff and puff with repetitive movements to burn off calories and fat but instead we work on fine-tuning the entire body, helping it to relaxed, vibrant, positive, health.

By working the entire body we stimulate the glands, which of course can help energize a sluggish metabolism. As the body's health improves you will find that your appetite becomes naturally controlled as your appetite-regulating system works better. You will start to eat less and change to healthier foods. It is difficult to believe but yoga actually does change your taste buds.

Most people find that gradually over the years their weight normalizes with continued yoga practice and it does lead people to start considering their diet. Doctors now tell us that the overload of toxins, chemicals, E numbers, and preservatives in our food can contribute to poor general health. People start feeling better and focusing on their health and this leads them into a brand new way of eating. Some pupils, however, have been steeped in bad eating habits for so long that they need a lot of guidance before change can be effected. We look at diet in more detail in Chapter 5.

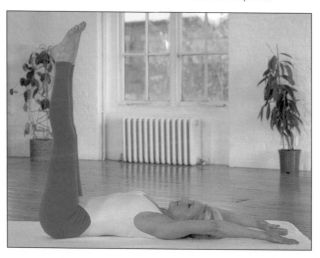

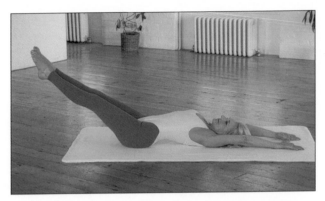

Yoga's slow stretches give the muscles a beautiful long, lean, toned shape – these weigh less than muscles toned by muscle-building exercise systems. All this will result in a gradual, natural, and healthy return to the best shape possible for your body type for life.

> "Let your food be your medicine; let your medicine be your food."
> Hypocrites

6 The Secret of Deep Relaxation and Meditation

One of the main reasons for our survival as a species is our incredible "fight or flight" response to sudden danger. Our bodies react immediately: the mind is filled with fear; adrenaline is secreted; blood sugar is raised; the blood supply to the muscles increases; muscles tense up; the blood-clotting mechanism goes up to enable the body to heal faster in case of wounds; breathing becomes rapid and shallow; the brain becomes hyper alert; the digestion is suppressed;

sexual desire is suppressed; blood vessels tighten to enable blood to flow through them faster and blood pressure is raised; the immune system is suppressed; more oxygen is consumed and more carbon dioxide is expelled. Humans, then, are programmed to look and be alert for more danger. In normal times a huge percentage of cellular energy goes into building new cells. However, during the fight or flight response instead it pours energy into the muscles with a result that tissue breakdown can eventually occur.

This reaction is brilliant if we have to run or fight. We need this reaction to sudden danger as it gives us the incredible extra power and energy we need to react in an emergency. Nowadays sudden danger is relatively rare, but the body's reaction to a stressful event continues and, whereas we all have to be grateful to it for our survival as a species, now this reaction can be the cause of major health problems due to the modern-day overload of mental stresses.

Doctors now realize that many diseases are caused by stress. The problem is that the body still reacts in this same way to the normal everyday stresses; the list is endless and is quite simply called "life". The stress reaction, if not balanced by periods of relaxation can now start to weaken the body and may give rise to such things as menstrual problems, high blood pressure, chronic fatigue, gastric ulcer, lower disease resistance, frequent headaches, cancer, and heart attacks. Unless we make a conscious effort to control our stress levels it is easy to let the stress response take hold. This is why yoga does us so much good and helps us live comfortably and easily in today's high-pressure world.

Yoga's wonderful stretches release the chronic tension that is held within our body. By deep breathing in every posture we stimulate life-giving oxygen to every cell and the act of slow, deep breathing calms our mind and aids deep relaxation. By concentrating on the balancing movements we take our mind off its troubles allowing it to calm down and feel peaceful. Relaxing at the end of yoga practice allows the stresses of the day to gently float away and frequent practice of meditation gives inner peace. As a result, the mind becomes clearer and calmer, muscular tension decreases, secretion of adrenaline is lowered, and breathing slows down. The heart rate slows, blood pressure normalizes and the blood-clotting mechanism is gently reduced, sweating gently ceases and the body becomes cooled and calmed, and digestion and the immune systems are relaxed and restored to normal.

> **"Our greatest experiences are our quietest moments."**
> Nietzsche (1844-1900)

7 The Secret of Radiant Health

These days everything comes with a manual – 60 pages just on the use of a mobile phone, 100 pages with a recipe book for your food mixer, a large manual for your washing machine, and a huge manual for your car. The most complex and brilliant system in your house, however, is your own body and sadly we are born without a manual!

If we did have one to instruct us on how to keep the body in perfect condition and this was taught to us at school, wouldn't that be a joy? We would then know how to care for all our body's complex systems and keep them in perfect condition. We would know how to oil our joints to keep them flexible, how to move our spine in all six directions to prevent it becoming stiff and aching,

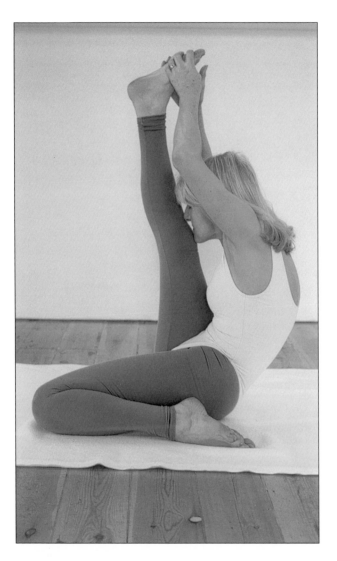

and we would practice weight-bearing movements to strengthen our bones. We would learn to eat correctly and never too much so that we never overload our stomach, heart, lungs, joints, and internal organs. We would then eat foods with health and vitality in mind rather than filling our bodies with junk and toxins that our bodies have no use for and find it difficult to remove.

We would learn the necessity of beautiful fresh air and correct breathing to make full use of our lungs and absorb more oxygen into our system. We would learn movements to get rid of tightness in our chest and calm our mind with slow and relaxing breathing.

We would learn how to keep our digestive system in good shape and the importance of movements to massage the digestive system such as the abdominal lift and contractions, the spinal twists and upwards stretch, and forwards and backwards bend. We would learn the effect of stress on the digestive system and realize the importance of relaxation to release the adverse effects of tension on our digestive organs.

Fight or Flight

We would learn to care for our heart and blood vessels. Under stress the body tries to make an enormous amount of energy available to enable us to flee or fight. This accelerates the heart rate and also squeezes the arteries and veins to try to raise the rate at which the blood flows through and as a result the blood pressure is raised. The clotting mechanism of the blood is also raised as the body sensibly thinks that if one has to flee or fight there could be wounds.

The net result of this is the heart pumps the thickened blood faster through narrow tubes. Because of this pressure, when the body is under long-term stress the arterial walls frequently become damaged. As the body tries its hardest to repair itself no matter how badly we treat it, it sends blood platelets and fatty acids to seal the damage; this, however, results in narrowing the arteries further. Continued stress increases the clotting mechanism and if a clot forms it can easily block a narrowed blood vessel and, of course, this can be fatal. So if we learn to stretch away our tensions daily, eat a healthy diet, and relax and allow our arteries and blood-clotting mechanism to calm down, the flee and fight reaction subsides, the blood-clotting mechanism is lowered, the arteries relax, and the blood pressure returns to normal. This would result in excellent care of our heart and circulatory system.

Our ductless glands control the amazing chemistry of our bodies, carefully regulating and controlling the mind–body relationship. If only our body manual taught us that the detrimental effect of stress could upset our entire glandular system!

The pituitary is the master gland of the body that controls the secretions of all the other glands. In yoga we help balance it with the Headstand. The thyroid gland controls our metabolism and the parathyroids control the calcium and phosphate level in the blood. The sex hormones, if imbalanced, can lead to menstrual problems and infertility in women and fertility problems in men. The Locust (see card 28) and Deep Relaxation (see card 10) poses help these areas tremendously.

The adrenal glands produce adrenalin to arouse the body to flee or fight, together with sex hormones and corticosteroids. Deep relaxation and meditation also relieve the stress that arouses this reaction. The pancreas is essential for the production of insulin to

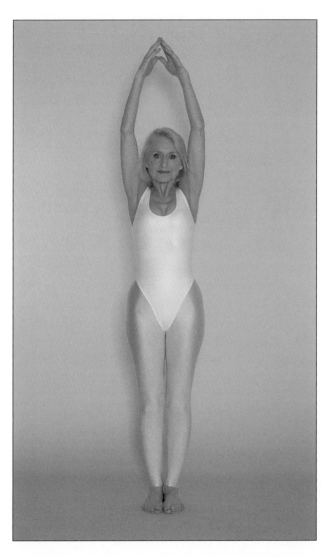

regulate the blood sugar of the body. Spinal twists help balance this organ and again a healthy natural diet stops overloading the body with excess sugar.

And, finally, we could learn how to control our nervous system and realize the incredible importance of our brain and spinal cord. The calming effect of the yoga movements also balances the involuntary symptoms of the flight-and-fight reaction, calming and cooling the body so reducing the adverse effects of chronic stress.

This book is your manual! Use it to learn ways of looking after your body, exercising it, eating fresh natural foods, breathing correctly, learning to relax and cope with stress, concentrating your mind on what you want rather than what you don't want, and keeping your joints and spine flexible and tension-free. In 15 minutes per day you will make the discovery of the secret of health and vitality forever, discovered over 5000 years ago. It is and always will be YOGA.

The Ancient Knowledge of Yoga

"Restraint, observance, posture, breath-control, sense withdrawal, concentration, meditative-absorption and enstasy are the eight members of yoga. Non-harming, truthfulness, non-stealing, chastity and greedlessness are the restraints."

Patanjali's *Yoga Sutras II*, 29–30

2
chapter

It is unclear when yoga actually originated, but seals were discovered depicting a yoga posture during the excavation of some ruins in prehistoric India in an area that now lies in Pakistan. These ruins revealed a very advanced civilization dating to around 5000 BC.

The earliest texts mentioning yoga were the Vedas, and these seem to have spanned about 2000 years, from 3000–1200 BC. These texts were followed by the Upanishads, written between 800 and 400 BC. The word "Upanishad" literally describes a sitting where the master or guru instructs his pupils. This is how yoga has been passed on from generation to generation, over the years. The spirit of the Upanishads can be compared with that of the New Testament: "The Kingdom of God is within you."

The Bhagavad Gita, dating from about 500 BC, tells of the struggle of the human soul, helping it to find God in all things and all things in God. It tells of a great battle for the rule of a Kingdom or the Kingdom of the soul, a battle between the forces of light and darkness. It shows that this is a battle that affects us all.

Patanjali's *Yoga Sutras*, written between 200 BC and AD 200, are another crucial yoga text. Patanjali wrote of a practical eight-part approach to yoga, frequently referred to as the Eight Limbs of Yoga.

These eight limbs were not regarded as a ladder to be climbed one rung at a time, but more the necessary ingredients in the recipe for life. The ancient yogis realized that life can be a difficult and complicated journey but its careful teachings and disciplines guide us along our path. They had a deep understanding of man's nature and of the mind–body connection, and they devised this system to help us obtain happiness and peace of mind, as well as a perfectly toned healthy body.

The Eight Limbs of Yoga

1 Yamas

These are guidelines necessary for our moral conduct and are the basic principles of right living and restraint; they include no violence, stealing, or envy and they command us to be truthful with both others and ourselves. Yoga teaches us that happiness is not in external objects but within ourselves and that the spirit of God is within each one of us.

2 Niyamas

These are the personal disciplines of daily life. They are cleanliness of mind and body, purity, contentment, study, work, and devotion to God or the universal spirit. Yoga teaches us that the body is the temple of the spirit and keeping the body in perfect condition is our duty.

3 Asanas

These are the yoga exercises or postures. It is said that there are 840,000 of them! These movements work the entire body, freeing it from tension, toning, firming, and strengthening every muscle,

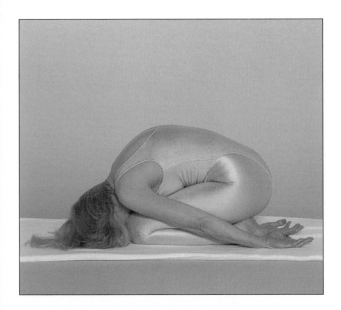

internal organ, and gland. The balancing postures teach us the power of concentration and focus, deep relaxation calms the mind and rids the body of chronic tension, and meditation trains the mind to achieve stillness and peace.

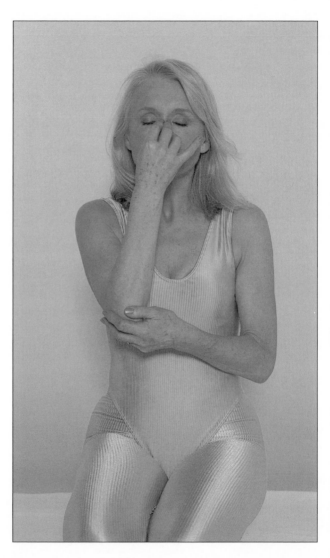

4 Pranayama

This is yoga's breath control. There are many breathing exercises in yoga to stimulate life-giving oxygen to reach every cell, to energize the body, and calm and soothe the mind. The word "pranayama" means "controlling the energy flow". Yoga teaches us how to use our breathing to control our life.

5 Pratyahara

This is the withdrawal of the senses from the external world to the self within to give one peace and calm. This is achieved by practicing the asanas and pranayama. Most of our daily activities necessitate our concentration and involvement with external objects and thoughts, but by concentrating on our body as we do the movements, and by concentrating on our breathing, the mind and body become peaceful and calm.

6 Dharana

This is the power of constant concentration and focusing of the mind. The mind is like the rays of the sun. When spread over a wide surface, the rays will be warming, but concentrate the rays and they become powerful enough to burn. Yoga balances start us on this path. They discipline the mind to concentrate on just one spot while performing the balances. This skill develops so that eventually one is able to concentrate and focus on a subject of interest even in the midst of turmoil.

7 Dhyama

This is meditation. Meditation is a powerful tool for freeing our minds from the pressures of life, helping us feel peaceful and calm. When this is accomplished, new ideas appear and the way ahead looks clearer.

8 Samadhi

This is the result of our total efforts and is the experience of enlightenment and bliss, living in the present moment, and the realization that we can manifest whatever we wish. The mind becomes full of joy and peace. It is the state of union with the universal spirit or God.

Another very important yoga text is the Hatha Yoga Pradipika, written by Svatmarama in the sixteenth century. The legend of the origin of yoga is as follows:

> **"Goddess Parvati, the wife of Lord Siva approached her Lord – the seed of all knowledge – for guidance to ease all the sufferings of humanity. Lord Siva then revealed to her the greatest of all sciences for the holistic development of man – the science of hatha yoga."**
> B.K.S. Iyengar

This knowledge was then passed on from guru to pupil until, eventually, Svatmarama wrote it down in the Pradipika. Hatha Yoga is the yoga most commonly practiced in the West today. It is the physical aspect of yoga. The aim is to perfect the health of the body and mind by physical exercises, balances, deep relaxation, meditation and breath control, and dietary observances.

> "Anyone who actively practices yoga be he young, old, or even very old, sickly or weak, can become a siddha [obtain yoga benefits and powers]. Anyone who practices can acquire siddhis, but not he who is lazy. Yoga siddhis are not obtained by merely reading textbooks. Nor are they reached by wearing yoga garments, or by conversations about yoga, but only through tireless practice. This is the secret of success. There is no doubt about it."
>
> Hatha Yoga Pradipika Ch4, v64–66

Meditation and Visualization

"The cure for all the illness of life is stored in the inner depth of life itself. The access to which becomes possible when we are alone. This solitude is a world in itself, full of wonders and resources within it. It is absurdly near, yet so inappropriately distant."

Rabindranath Tagore

Meditation

We have now fully discussed yoga's wonderful system of exercises, breathing, balances, healthy eating, and deep relaxation. All this leads to a beautiful youthful body, energy, and a tremendous feeling of wellbeing. Living in today's high-pressure world, however, can be exceedingly difficult, full of highs and lows, moments of tension, deep-seated anxiety, insecurity, frustration, struggle, noise, and work overload, etc, all of which can lead to inner turmoil which can adversely affect both the body and mind. We try to sort ourselves out by resorting to the usual remedies – drinking strong coffee and other stimulants to give us more energy, alcohol to help us relax, and sleeping pills to calm our overactive brains and help us to sleep. This only works on the symptoms, not the cause of the problem. The cause is our inability to still our brain and make it calm and serene, and the overload of stimuli can result in chronic stress that can eventually lead to disease.

The amazing thing is that well over 5000 years ago the yogis of ancient India realized that by learning to calm the mind we can help ourselves to a feeling of calm and peace and by so doing alleviate the damaging effects of stress on the body and mind. Calming the mind however is difficult and, like the yoga exercises, quite simply gets better with practice. There are many techniques and because we are all different it is vital to find the method that works best for you. These techniques are collectively referred to as meditation.

How to Meditate

- Sit in a comfortable position with your back straight. The lotus position is ideal but by no means essential and if you are not yet comfortable in it then a crossed-leg position, kneeling position, or your favorite armchair will do fine.
- Make sure that you are warm enough as your temperature can drop a little during meditation.
- Make sure that you will not be disturbed.
- If you have an appointment later, it is wise to set an alarm clock for your allocated meditation time, as it is not unusual to fall asleep during your first attempts at meditation.
- Now close your eyes and concentrate on your breathing. Don't try to change it or regulate it, just bring your attention to it.
- If your mind wanders, and it does even for experienced meditators, just bring your attention back to your breathing. Please don't think that you are bad at meditating if your mind wanders, just relax and gently bring your mind back to your breathing and allow all other thoughts to just slip away.

The above technique is my preferred method of meditation. Other ways include focusing on a special object like a beautiful flower or leaf, a special piece of crystal or rock, a candle flame (make sure that it is safe

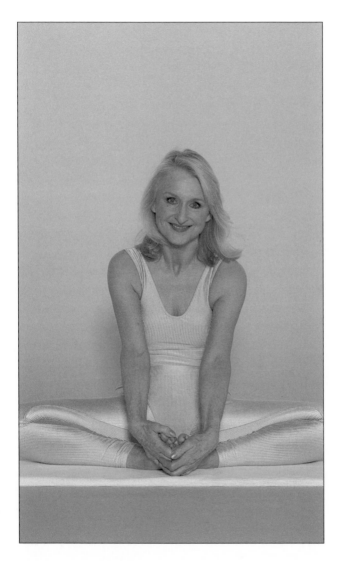

if you are liable to fall asleep), or a religious symbol. Literally any single object that works for you is fine. Some people prefer to repeat a mantra. Choose a word like peace or calm or the yoga word "om" pronounced "aum." This word is sacred to yoga and means "what was, what is and what shall be". Take a deep breath in and as you exhale say it softly and slowly making your exhalation and the sound last as long as possible, then repeat it over and over again until a feeling of peace flows through you.

Start with 10 minutes of meditation if you can and gradually increase it to 20 minutes. Do your meditation at a time to suit your own schedule. Early morning is traditionally a good time for meditation, but if your house is in chaos then just choose a time when you can relax and enjoy the peace and calm it will give you.

When the mind is thinking hard it is busy and frequently overloaded with worries about the past and anxieties about the future, the brain in this state emits rapid beta brain waves. Once we start to calm the mind and focus on one object or our breathing, the mind stays in the present tense, which is fine and free from stressful thoughts. When this feeling of calm and peace flows through our being the brain starts to emit slower and more rhythmic alpha-style brain waves. This lovely peaceful sense of calm pervades our whole being, breathing slows down, stress hormone levels and blood pressure fall and meditators find that they are less prone to stress and depression, they also have more energy, need less sleep, and look younger and more radiant then non-meditators.

> **"These days everybody wants Botox. I have had it myself only twice – since the meditation I don't need it."**
> Jeya Prakash, Consultant plastic surgeon, based in Harley Street

Don't Expect Instant Results

One of the problems of meditation for Westerners is that nothing much happens at first. You find it difficult to switch off and wonder if it is doing you any good. Please persevere. Meditation does require practice and you will benefit from all your meditations and eventually you will feel very clear, calm, and focused and frequently you will receive new and clear insight into a particular area of your life and problems will seem easier to solve. Please don't begrudge the time taken for meditation as you are always more productive and proactive after meditation than before.

By meditating we are not trying to find peace and calm, they are already within us. We are trying to get rid of the incredible overload of mental stimuli to enable us to give our natural peace a place in our hectic lives.

Sometimes it is very difficult to switch off and at times like these we need to adopt a detached attitude and relax, realizing that this is the present moment just as it is. Meditation, like everything else in life, requires practice. You will benefit from all your meditations, although some will be more relaxing than others. The relaxing effect will stay with you for quite a while so try to meditate for a number of short periods of time every day – even five minutes is fine. You will find your overall stress levels reduce dramatically and your mind will become clear, calm, energized, and focused.

Once you have been meditating for a while you may experience a beautiful relaxed and thought-free feeling – this is known as "going into the gap." As you continue to meditate this will become more frequent. Here you experience contact with the universal spirit which gives us access to unlimited intelligence, you then stop relying on the opinion of others and become guided from within, you realize that you manifest your own destiny and experience a beautiful inner joy and confidence, and nothing is impossible for you. Things don't seem to worry you as much, you learn to trust your own gut instincts which, of course, are the real you, and frequently when your mind is calm new ideas and solutions to problems just arrive out of the blue. All this results in a lovely feeling of deep inner peace and self-confidence.

Things will still go wrong – the cleaners will still ruin your best suit, you will still get held up in traffic. The problems of daily life will not go away, but deep down inside you don't worry as much because you learn to accept them as part of life. You stay calm and focused on your goals and regard the hassles of life as almost necessary hurdles and challenges on life's amazing journey and no matter what happens you can still look at a beautiful flower or tree and just be happy in spite of it all.

On a purely cosmetic basis there is simply nothing that will erase your lines and wrinkles more than meditation – again I quote from the respected leading Consultant cosmetic plastic surgeon Jeya Prakash:

> **"At home I practice meditation for 20 minutes every day. After 5 minutes of my mantra, the stress goes out of my head and I have a few minutes of completely static pure mind. Meditation is like washing your body from the inside. I follow it with 10 minutes of yoga. People say I look fresher, more vibrant. This is the real secret of youthful skin."**
> Jeya Prakash

I totally agree. Your face is a reflection of how you are inside, if you want to get rid of a sagging, tense face – cleanse, tone, and nourish from within.

The Power of Visualization

Once the mind is quiet and calmed by deep breathing, yoga exercises, and meditation, we can then learn to control our minds and discipline them to create and enjoy our heart's desires. This power is not unusual, we are in fact using it every moment of every day: it is the power of our imagination. Yoga however teaches us to take control and use this incredible power to our own advantage.

In this way we can learn to create a fabulous life and a fantastic future and fill our lives with health, happiness, hope, and creativity instead of filling our minds with lack, fear, limitations, worry, and difficulty.

We are creating our own lives by the thoughts we habitually think. When we imagine something, we create an idea or a mental picture or a sense of something. By learning to discipline our minds we can learn to create for ourselves in our own minds a very clear picture of what we would like to manifest in our lives. Now by stilling our minds and concentrating on that image at least three times per day we start to make the image appear very real in our lives. As we concentrate on the end product we start to get excited about our image – this gives it more positive creative energy until the thing we just pictured is achieved. This power can be used to create anything in your life from better health, a better body, a new job, better relationships, to more money or quitting bad habits.

When you learn to quieten the mind and focus on your goal at least three times a day and, every day, you will find the plan is permanently in your mind and regardless of limitations, money, time, difficulties, it will be achieved.

> "When you are inspired by some great purpose, some extraordinary project, all your thoughts break their bonds, your mind transcends limitation, your consciousness expands in every direction and you find yourself in a new great and wonderful world. Dormant forces, faculties and talents become alive and you discover yourself to be a greater person by far than you have ever imagined yourself to be."
>
> Patanjali
>
> Yoga Sutras

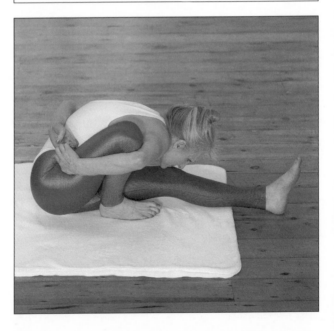

How Power Visualization Works

Our master teachers through the ages have always known that our thoughts determine our destiny.

> "Ask and it will be given to you, seek and you will find, knock and it will be opened unto you."
>
> Matthew 7.7

> "If thou canst believe, all things are possible to him that believeth."
>
> Mark 9.23

> "What we vividly imagine, ardently desire, enthusiastically act upon, must inevitably come to pass."
>
> Colin P Sisson

> "If one advances confidently in the direction of his dreams, and endeavours to live the life which he has imagined he will meet with a success unexpected in common hours."
>
> Henry David Thoreau

> "The greatest discovery of my generation is that human beings can alter their lives by altering their attitudes of mind."
>
> William James

> "Your mind will be like its habitual thoughts, for the soul becomes dyed with the colour of its thoughts."
>
> Marcus Aurelius 5.16

> "I am responsible for what I see, I choose the feelings I experience and I decide upon the goal that I would achieve and everything that seems to happen to me I ask for and receive as I have asked."
>
> *A course in Miracles*

Nowadays our scientific experts seek to explain this by teaching us that we are all, along with everything else in the universe, composed of a force of energy and are all part of one huge vibrating energy field. As human beings we are extremely fortunate to be equipped with an incredible nervous system and thought process enabling us to make changes in our lives simply by changing the thoughts we think. Thoughts are also energy vibrations that are magnetic and attract and create things in our

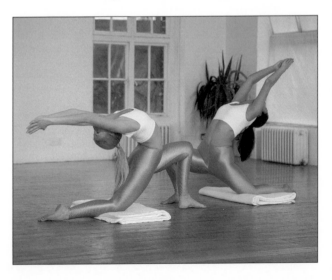

lives. By changing our thoughts and, by so doing, changing our energy field, we can then create changes in the wider energy field and so can start to make positive changes in our own lives and eventually can manifest our own destiny. These changes can be brought about by the power of thought. Putting it simply, whatever you put your attention and intention on will grow stronger in your life and whatever you take your attention and intention off will grow weaker and gradually disappear.

> "Inherent in every intention and desire is the mechanics for its fulfilment. Intention and desire in the field of pure potentiality have infinite organising power. And when we increase an intention in the fertile ground of pure potentiality we put this infinite organising power to work for us."
> Deepak Chopra

We can now see how yoga – the union between body, mind, and spirit – works so well for us. By creating an excellent healthy body with your yoga exercises, energizing and calming the mind with the deep breathing, increasing the power of concentration and focus by performing the balances, and learning one-point focus and calm in the meditation our minds are then perfectly equipped for us to put our clear desires into the energy field.

This brilliant technique can be used to create anything we desire! I know it all sounds just too simple and your logical brain comes back with at least 50 reasons why it won't work. But never forget that great thinkers have always thought of the outcome of their

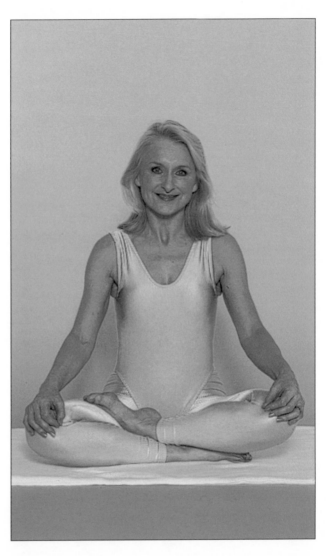

desires and not the hurdles on their path. Once you start thinking in this way and putting your desires in a clear concise way, writing them down and putting them into your thoughts at least three times a day with calm serenity and total belief in the outcome you desire, you will find that your dreams are fulfilled with effortless ease.

> **"If you have faith as a grain of mustard seed, nothing shall be impossible unto you."**
> Matthew 7.20

But if your mind constantly thinks about the worries, troubles, and obstacles in your path of life, then these will manifest in your life.

> **"The thing which I greatly feared is come upon me and that which I was afraid of is come unto me."**
> Job 3.25

Once we learn this amazing power of the human mind and refuse to think of the obstacles in our path, we can then focus on our goals with calm, peace, and serenity knowing that the thing we desire will manifest in our lives.

> **"Whosoever shall say unto this mountain, 'be thou removed, and be thou cast into the sea' and shall not doubt in his heart, but shall believe that these things which he saith shall come to pass, he shall have whatsoever he saith."**
> Mark 11.23

The last quote, I believe, is one of the most powerful quotes of all time. Our mountains are our troubles, difficulties, inferiorities, and negative thought patterns. Once you believe that your mountains or difficulties can be overcome and focus on the outcome or goal of your dreams, your life can change.

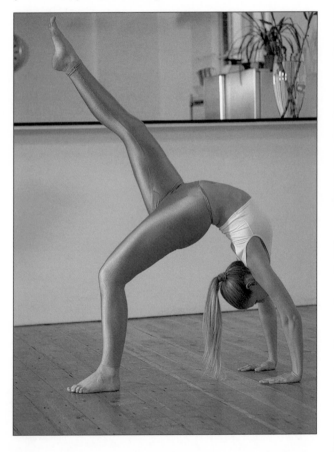

How to Use this Wonderful Power

First decide what you would like. This might sound crazy but most people will say with a grin, "Oh I don't know, a better life, or more money, etc." You must be specific. Say, for example, you wanted to drive your car from London to Inverness. You would need a road map, a car in good condition, probably a place to stay en route to break your journey, adequate money for your petrol and food for the journey, and sufficient time to complete the journey. This is just simple planning but without it you won't get there. Now your life is your journey and you must be specific.

- Where do you want to go in life?
- What do you want to achieve?
- Where do you want to live?
- How do you want to look?
- How healthy and fit do you want to be?
- How much money do you want to earn?
- What places would you like to visit?
- What car would you like to drive?
- What job would you like to have?
- What would be the house of your dreams?
- How many children would you like to have?
- What hobbies would you like to take up?

If you have never answered these questions before, sit down in a quiet place for about half an hour and just answer each one honestly and calmly without limits. Make sure you do this regardless of your age, present position, etc. Now you have your road map for your life.

1 Now put the five most important goals on a card in a brief form in the present tense, for example: "I am a very fit and healthy architect earning $200,000 per year. I live in a beautiful old house in the country with my wife and two children." Make sure that the picture you have described represents your ideal picture of your ideal life.

2 Carry this card with you and look at it at least three times per day. On waking, before your meditation at lunch, and before bed.

3 By doing this you will start being the architect and your dream life will start to become a reality. Every day make sure you do something to help you achieve your goals.

4 Don't make your happiness in life dependent on the fulfillment of every part of your dream. Simply decide now to be happy, no matter what and to enjoy every part of your journey towards your dream.

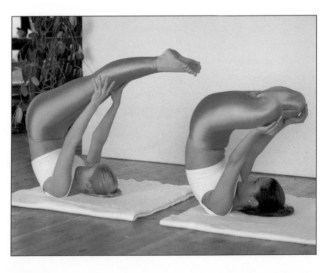

5 Believe that your dreams will be manifested, expect hurdles and challenges along the way, and be flexible. Sometimes on the way to a dream, something better turns up. Just believe that the great goodness that surrounds you has wonderful plans for you, sometimes better than your dreams.

In this way your dreams will gradually be fulfilled easily and effortlessly. Your subconscious mind will guide you, new ideas will start to flow, the roadblocks on the way to your dreams will gradually be overcome, and you will start to live the life that once was only in your dreams.

> "Mind is the master power that moulds and makes.
> And we are mind and evermore we take the tool of thought and shaping what we will
> Bring forth a thousand joys or a thousand ills.
> We think in secret and it comes to pass
> Our world is but our looking glass."
>
> James Allen, *As a Man Thinketh*

Salutation to the Dawn
Look to this day!
For it is life, the very life of life
In its brief course lie all the verities and realities of your existence.
The bliss of growth
The glory of action
The splendour of achievement
For yesterday is but a dream
And tomorrow is only a vision
But today well lived makes yesterday a dream of happiness
And every tomorrow a vision of hope
Look well therefore to this day
Such is the salutation to the dawn.   Kalidasa

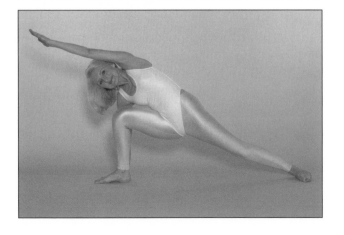

Yoga Today

The collective knowledge of these ancient texts began to appear in the West at the end of the nineteenth century and since then interest in yoga has grown and today it is at an all-time high. Students of all ages are pouring into classes to learn yoga, and for many diverse reasons. Some come simply to improve their body shape, some to cure an aching back, some to relieve stress. Whatever the reason, yoga can help you live healthily in this chaotic, exciting, and wonderful modern world.

While Hatha yoga remains the most widely practiced form of yoga in the West, other forms include:

- Raja Yoga – the yoga of the mind;
- Karma Yoga – the yoga of action;
- Bhakti Yoga – the yoga of devotion;
- Jhana Yoga – the yoga of the intellect.

Because of the many approaches to teaching yoga, finding a class to suit you can be very confusing. I often receive phone calls from people inquiring as to what sort of yoga I teach. I suppose that since I have been teaching for over 30 years, by now I have put my individual stamp on the ancient art. Throughout this time, I have tried to make yoga understandable, enjoyable, and available to everyone. It is my firm belief that everyone can benefit tremendously from yoga practice.

But how can you find a class that will be to your liking? I am afraid that this will be a bit like trying to find everything else – from a builder to a hairdresser. Often you have to try several until the perfect one appears. There are some excellent yoga teachers around, quite simply search for a class until you find one that works for you. As a first move, you can't do better than look in your local newspaper or ask in your local library to find classes running near where you live.

Guidelines for Practicing Yoga

You need very little equipment for your yoga practice so it is easy to fit in with any lifestyle. Once you have learnt your basic movements you can do them at home or on holiday. Your yoga will go with you wherever you go. Having said this, there are a few basic guidelines that you should take note of before you start.

- You need a warm airy room if you are practicing inside, but in warmer climates it is wonderful to do your yoga in the fresh air in the warmth of the early morning or evening. Never practice in the heat of direct sun.

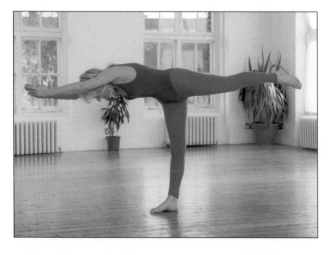

- You need a mat or blanket to sit on. My preference is for a blanket or thick warm mat for internal practice. However, if you are practicing yoga outside, perhaps on a beach, you need a waterproof mat to keep you clean and dry.

- Wear loose clothing, ideally a leotard and leggings for women, or leggings and a close fitting t-shirt. Jogging bottoms or shorts and a t-shirt are best for men. If you are outdoors in a warm climate, your swimsuit is just fine.

- Bare feet are essential for yoga practice.

- Always wait at least two hours after a main meal before you practice yoga.

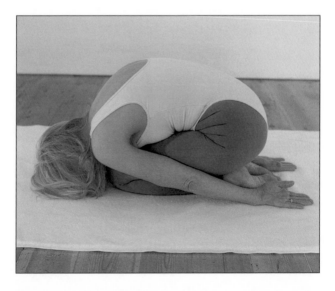

- The golden rule of yoga is never, ever to strain. Don't worry if you are stiff and unco-ordinated to start with. This is quite normal. Just persevere, work at your own pace and you will be delighted at how quickly your body responds to the movements and how much more flexible you are after only a few weeks of practice. You will start to feel better almost immediately and will soon be delighted with your new svelte shape.

- Although yoga is for everyone, if you have any health concerns it is always wise to check with your doctor before you begin.

- Although yoga is good for your health and some movements are particularly beneficial for certain conditions, never substitute yoga for your doctor's treatment.

- If you are pregnant and have not done any yoga before, then please wait until after your check-up at about 15 weeks. If everything is OK and your doctor is happy, then you may start to practice yoga very gently, omitting any movements marked unsuitable for pregnancy.

- Wait until after your six-week check-up following the baby's birth before you recommence your yoga practice. If your doctor is happy for you to recommence your yoga practice, then inform your teacher of the nature of your delivery. Go gently, and you will soon find your shape and energy coming back fast.

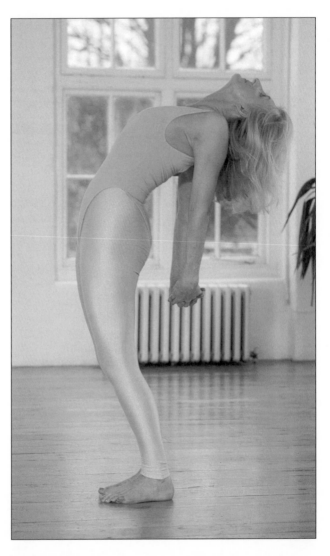

- In yoga, we breathe deeply with every movement to help to stimulate oxygen to reach every cell, and energize our entire systems. Breathing is done through the nose. As a general rule, gently allow your abdominals to push out as you inhale deeply through the nose at the start of a posture and exhale slowly and quietly through the nose as you go into the movement. While in the positions, breathe calmly and peacefully through the nose.

Yoga for Complete Health

"**Make the most of yourself for that is all there is of you.**"

Ralph Waldo Emerson

In this chapter, we look at aspects of yoga beyond the exercises. I do hope that by now I have whetted your appetite and you can't wait to get started. Yoga is the most wonderful system for promoting positive health and wellbeing. Its brilliant combination of amazing exercises, balancing postures, breathing techniques, deep relaxation, meditation, and visualization, together with a healthy diet, will help you to radiant health and vitality for many years to come. I hope you come to love it as much as I do.

Enjoy your yoga!

Yoga and Diet

If you have already started practicing the postures in this book, I hope you will have found that your flexibility is getting better, you have more energy, your shape is improving, and you are finding it easier to cope with life's many challenges.

All these benefits and many others start to appear, sometimes as if out of the blue. Many subtle changes occur in your body and often this prompts people to question their diet.

Once you start feeling good about yourself you stop wanting to harm your body; junk foods that you may have once referred to as "treats" may not have the same appeal and eventually you will regard them as toxins. This is yoga's way of naturally encouraging

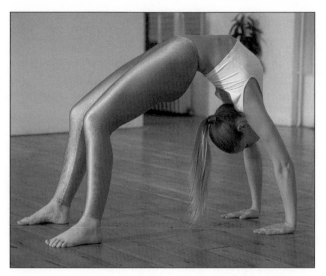

you to eat foods that are beneficial to your body and that enhance the prana or life-force within you.

As yoga continues to stimulate this flow of positive health within you, you will notice other changes happening. It is likely that your tastes will alter, you will go off foods and drinks that you once thought you couldn't live without. You start to listen to your body. It is usual for my pupils to admit that before they took up yoga they would regularly enjoy a heavy meal washed down with two or three glasses of wine, but that nowadays their preference is for a lighter, fresher meal with one glass of wine or none at all. This is the best and most natural way to lose weight and cultivate leanness, positive health, and vitality.

The more you progress in yoga, the more these changes are effected from within, but a lot of my pupils are keen to hurry things along. They see their shape changing due to the exercises and ask me for dietary advice. They want results now! This is why I set out below my own eating plan that has helped thousands of my students.

Over 40 years ago, as part of my nursing training, I had the good fortune to work on a ward specializing in nutritional and metabolic problems and eating disorders. This gave me a lifelong interest in nutrition. I realized that if we ate fresh, healthy foods in as natural a state as possible, our bodies would glow with positive health and wellbeing. I understood that whatever diet we choose, it must fit in with our lifestyle and cope with our social and work commitments. Also, it must be well balanced to give us all the nutrients we need to keep us slim and healthy and to provide us with energy.

I designed my plan when my own weight fluctuations and lack of energy made me listen to the experts with whom I was working. Over the years, I have adapted the plan to fit in with changes in my own life, as well as integrating the knowledge I have since gained about yoga and nutrition. However, the basic plan is still very much the same – simple, fresh, healthy food in the correct quantities to maintain our weight easily and effortlessly, and, most importantly, to keep us healthy and give us energy.

Back in the Stone Age, man's diet would have consisted of fresh fruits, vegetables, meat, and fish. In those days there was no processed, canned, or packaged food, no fast food, and no quick "heat and serve" meals. Early man had no insecticides, additives, preservatives, or E numbers to contend with. This was all brought home to me when I presented doctors with the results of tests on my patients in the nutrition ward where I was working. In the ward there was one lady with a severe eating disorder and no treatment

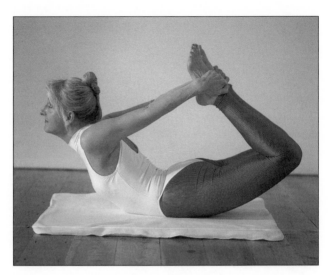

had been of help. I mentioned to the doctors that I had seen junk food and drink being smuggled to her by visiting relatives on many occasions – maybe this should be taken into consideration. One doctor suddenly said, "Barbara, if we all ate simple food in as fresh and natural a state as possible, so many of these problems and disorders could be eliminated."

I will remember those words for the rest of my life because, until that moment, I had thought of my nutritional work as something only relating to my patients, but when I thought of my own health, everything seemed to click into place. So, I designed my fabulous natural food plan and reaped the wonderful benefits. I am glad that I learnt so young!

I am not going to list all the vitamins and their benefits – that information is available everywhere. But it is vital to understand that although canned and frozen fruits and vegetables can be shown to have the same amount of vitamins as fresh produce, they lack the essence called "prana" or life-force contained in fresh fruits and vegetables. This cannot be seen or measured but, believe me, it is there!

Secrets of a Healthy Diet

1 Don't eat standing up

Obey this rule for one week and see the difference! So many people constantly nibble, eating on the go, eating between meals, eating the kids leftovers, "tasting" as they cook the dinner etc. This means that they are never really hungry and are always amazed when their skinny friends say, "I'm starving" and sit and eat a good meal. When you stop picking and nibbling your appetite will become fine-tuned and you will enjoy your food so much more. Everything tastes great when you are really hungry. You will also know exactly what you ate and stop kidding yourself that you eat like a bird.

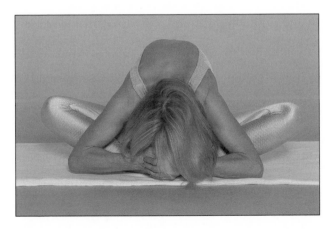

2 Never eat between meals

Again, a continuation of the rule above, this stops the constant nibbling and snacking. When you sit down and eat three meals a day calmly and slowly with nothing in between you will find it makes a huge difference to your weight and the way you feel. You will feel so much more in control!

> **"Never more than half fill your stomach with food, leave a quarter for fluid and a quarter for digestion."**
> Hatha Yoga Pradipika 4.58

This is brilliant advice from yoga's ancient texts. Now let's recap – if you don't eat standing up and don't eat between meals, you eat slowly and calmly, never more than half filling your stomach with food, you will normally find any excess weight slipping away naturally.

What to Eat

In yoga we eat for total positive health and for stimulating the "prana" or life-force within us. This is pure natural food. Prepare your meals from the following selections: feast on beautiful fresh fruit and natural healthy juices, fresh vegetables and salads, enjoy natural whole grains, nuts and seeds, a little milk, butter, cheese, natural organic live yogurt, eggs, moderate amounts of fish and chicken, and a small amount of red meat. Olive oil and walnut oil are excellent for inclusion in salad dressings with either lemon juice or vinegar and be sure to add fresh herbs and spices to flavor your food. Try to drink at least two liters of water per day and enjoy herbal tea and natural fruit juices. Try to restrict coffee and tea to a maximum of five cups per day and have decaffeinated if possible. Restrict alcohol to just one glass of wine a day if desired.

Avoid all diet products (they may contain additives and it is best to just eat fresh, natural, healthy food), cakes, sweets (candy), biscuits (cookies), chocolates, bagels, buns, pasta (apart from wholegrain), pizza, puddings and ice cream, packaged cereals (apart from organic whole grain ones), jam (jelly), sandwich spreads and fillers, fizzy drinks, and heat and serve meals. Keep the accent on fresh, fresh, fresh food – nothing canned, frozen, or preserved. (I have never seen a slim person asking for a diet drink or using sweeteners but I find my larger friends use diet products constantly.)

Think back to our Stone Age ancestors. They could only eat food that they could grow, catch, or trap – just a pure, natural, healthy diet. This is obviously the diet nature intended for us. And finally, my advice to you is make your own plans from the foods advised and

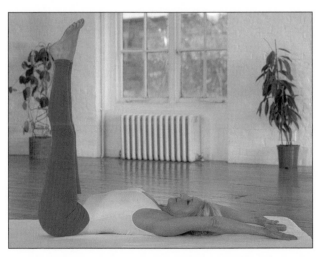

enjoy your food. If you find your weight not slipping away as you wish, simply cut down on your portions. I know it is hard but, if you are heavier than your ideal weight for your height and build, quite simply eating less will do the trick.

When you take time out to practice yoga movements and deep breathing, meditate and eat healthy foods, you will find that your overall health starts to improve dramatically. And as your health improves your health problems gradually lessen. Having said this, I still find pupils who wish to learn an exercise to help with a particular health problem! Ill health is a manifestation of imbalance within the body and although there are movements that are extremely beneficial for specific problems, there can be no short cut.

Your body needs daily exercise and 15 minutes of yoga will do just fine. You must also learn to relax during the day, even if you only take short breaks and totally relax in your office chair. Slow, deep breathing can be fitted in to the busiest day and it is especially beneficial if taken in fresh air. Use the power of visualization daily to visualize your whole body as radiant with vibrant, glowing, positive health.

Yoga also teaches us to listen to our symptoms, as these are the body's way of telling us that it is unhappy with its current treatment. Frequently, by making the necessary lifestyle changes, aches and pains start to melt away. But there are some routines that are of particular use when we are suffering from specific symptoms. In the table at the end of this chapter I give my favorite prescriptions for some of the most widespread modern maladies.

My Plan

Rules

- Eat three meals a day and nothing in between apart from the recommended drinks.
- Never eat standing up. Sit down and enjoy your food.
- Make your food look beautiful, garnish it with herbs, have flowers on the table or light scented candles in the evening.
- If you are out at a dinner party, don't offend your hosts by refusing their food. If an item is served that is not on your plan, then just accept a small portion. If you would like two glasses of wine during a special evening, then simply go without the previous evening.

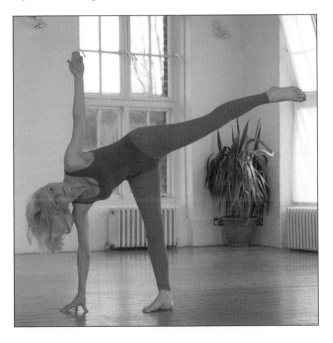

- If you are in a tremendous hurry and have no time for lunch or to prepare any of the items suggested, then:

  a) have 2 bananas – they are excellent for lunch when you are in a rush and are the most perfectly packaged "fast food," containing many essential vitamins and minerals;

  b) when at home, place 1 small carton of natural organic yogurt, 1 banana, 1 teaspoon of honey and 1 carton of raspberries in a blender and drink this for your lunch. This is fabulous – healthy, nutritious, and delicious!

- If one day you break your diet and eat some junk food, don't feel guilty and cut back the next day. Just accept the fact that you are human. Start back on the plan the next day.

[Note: I advise you to consult your doctor or nutritionist before starting on this or any other eating plan to make sure that it is suitable for your personal dietary requirements.]

PERMITTED FOODS

Fresh Fruit

One portion equals one of each of the following:

apple

$\frac{1}{2}$ small melon

pear

large slice of watermelon

orange

$\frac{1}{2}$ grapefruit

peach

3 apricots

small banana

3 plums

dish of berries

3 figs

These are only examples. All fresh fruit is allowed. Do not use canned, frozen, or stewed fruit.

Fresh vegetables and salads

All vegetables are allowed except crisps, chips (fries), potatoes, and corn on the cob. The latter two may be eaten occasionally as a substitute for rice and pasta for dinner. Try to have as much variety as possible. Have them raw, steamed, boiled, or stir-fried – never deep-fried. 1 portion = 3 tablespoons of cooked vegetables.

Salad ingredients

Have as much as you like but make sure the ingredients are fresh and raw. Only use 1 tablespoonful of dressing.

Fish

All varieties are allowed. Grill (broil), steam, poach, or pan fry with very little oil. Do not deep fry. Try to have oily fish three times a week.

Chicken, poultry, game, and veal

All varieties are allowed. Grill (broil), poach, steam, barbecue – do not deep fry.

Red meat

Beef, lamb, pork, venison, etc. Have no more than twice a week.

Eggs and cheese

Both are allowed in the amounts shown.

Grains

Only whole grains are allowed and in the amounts shown. No white bread, rice, or pasta.

Milk

Semi-skimmed (½ pint daily) and natural yogurt in the amounts indicated.

Not permitted – until you have reached your desired weight:

Bagels; hot chocolate; beer; ice cream; biscuits (cookies); jam (jelly); breakfast cereals; puddings; buns; soft drinks; cakes; spirits; canned drinks; sugar; chips (fries); sweets (candy); chocolates.

Avoid all additives and preservatives. Just eat natural healthy food.

BREAKFAST

Choose from:

1 portion fresh fruit and 1 natural yogurt;

2 portions of any fresh fruit chopped up, drizzled with 1 teaspoon of honey;

1oz of sliced hard cheese or 4oz cottage cheese with 1 sliced apple or pear;

1 slice granary toast with a little butter and either 1 piece of fresh fruit or a glass of fresh fruit juice;

1 poached egg on a slice of granary toast with a scraping of butter.

Plus tea or coffee from your allowance.

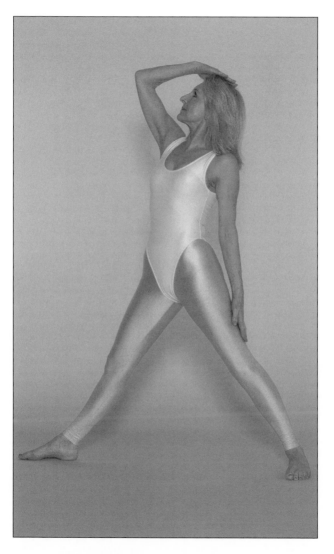

LUNCH

Choose from:

4oz chicken, turkey, or fish; or 2 eggs, 2oz cheese; or 4oz red meat (remember, red meat is allowed only twice a week) with large salad – use a variety of raw fresh ingredients to make your choice different every day, together with 1 tablespoon olive oil and vinegar dressing. Instead of salad, you may have 2 fresh-cooked vegetables;

1 sandwich made with 2 slices wholegrain bread and a scraping of butter or mayonnaise, filled with salad and 2oz of chicken, turkey, or fish, or 1 egg or 1oz cheese;

$\frac{1}{2}$ avocado pear filled with 3oz prawns, topped with 1 dessertspoon marie rose dressing or lemon mayonnaise and garnish with green salad;

1 Cesar salad using cos lettuce, 1 tablespoon dressing, $1\frac{1}{2}$ oz Parmesan cheese, and $\frac{1}{2}$ slice granary toast made into garlic croutons;

Salade Nicoise – lettuce, tomatoes, green beans (cooked), 5 black olives, 3oz tuna fish, and $\frac{1}{2}$ hard-boiled egg, with 1 tablespoon oil and vinegar dressing.

DINNER

Choose from:

Starter

melon;

fresh asparagus with a little butter or vinaigrette;

clear soup;

tomato salad;

mixed salad;

mini Cesar salad (without croutons).

Main Course

4oz chicken, fish, veal, or red meat (remember, red meat is allowed only twice a week);

small whole grain, rice, or pasta dish;

1 large bowl of mussels cooked in garlic, wine, and onions;

large platter of mixed grilled seafood including prawns, salmon, langoustine, and calamari;

plus 2 fresh vegetables or a large raw salad with 1 tablespoonful of oil and vinegar dressing.

Dessert

1 piece fresh fruit, plus tea or coffee from your allowance.

To drink

Six–eight glasses of water a day; herbal tea as desired; coffee and tea, preferably decaffeinated, no more than 5 cups a day; wine – 1 glass a day, with dinner if desired.

Copy this plan, slip it in your bag, and take it everywhere. There is plenty of choice in the plan, so it will fit into the busiest lifestyle and cope with any social engagement, but it is important to vary your diet to make sure you have all the vitamins and minerals you require. For instance, if you have chicken with salad for lunch, then have fish and vegetables for dinner.

By keeping to this plan, it is easily possible to lose 2–3 lbs a week. Once you have reached your desired weight, gradually increase the amount you eat until you find how much you need to maintain this weight. If you gain another 3–4 lbs, then immediately return to your plan until your weight is corrected. You will find that you gradually reach a level where your weight stays the same and you are able to maintain it effortlessly and naturally. Then you will keep in shape for life. If you are happy with your weight and just want to eat for excellent health, then follow the plan and increase the amounts of the foods in accordance with your taste and appetite.

Finally, I am often asked if I am a vegetarian, as is the preference of many yoga devotees. I have tried a vegetarian diet but, quite honestly, it does not suit me and I feel much better for including meat, fish, and chicken in my diet. The choice must be an individual one. Listen to your body and make a personal decision according to what feels right for you. Good luck and good health!

Yoga and Pregnancy

I recommend yoga practice throughout pregnancy. However, as the pregnancy progresses it is important to have your medical practitioner's go-ahead, as well as guidance from a trained yoga

15-Minute Yoga Box

teacher as movements have to be altered to cope with the increasing size of your baby. In general, if you have no history of miscarriage and have been practicing yoga regularly prior to becoming pregnant, there is no reason why you should not continue. Avoid all movements that put strain on the abdomen – the Pose of the Locust, the Salute to the Sun, the Pose of a Dog, the Pose of a Boat, Abdominal Lift, and Contractions are all forbidden, as are the Spinal Twists, the Shoulder Stand, and the Headstand. Yoga breathing and relaxation techniques are most beneficial. The Pose of a Cat is excellent for relieving lower back pain.

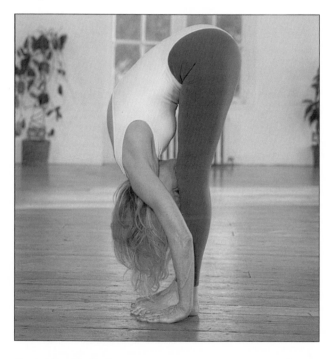

If you have never practiced yoga before and would like to start yoga in pregnancy, wait until after your 15th week of pregnancy. With your medical practitioner's permission and a good teacher, yoga will help both your pregnancy and labor. Enjoy your pregnancy, learn to relax, stay calm, and listen to beautiful music. Peaceful, relaxed mums make happy, calm babies.

[Note: Although yoga is extremely beneficial to your health, it must never be used as a substitute for treatment by a qualified medical practitioner. Before doing the recommended movements please ask your practitioner for permission and find a qualified yoga teacher to help and guide you.]

Exercises for Specific Health Problems

Health Problem	Exercise	Beneficial Effects
Arthritis and rheumatism	Start each day with a 15-minute Miracle	To keep the spine flexible
	Arm Exercises	Ensuring maximum flexibility in the shoulders
	Thigh Stretch	Helping your hips, knees, and ankles
Asthma	Start each day with a 15-minute Miracle	To relieve tension from the spine

	Alternate Nostril Breathing	Reduces stress levels.
	Backwards Bend	Helping to relieve tightness in the chest
Back problems	Start each day with a 15-minute Miracle	Flexibility in the spine
	Pose of a Cat	To relieve tension from spine
	Pose of a Boat	To soothe the spine
Tension and headaches	Chest Expansion Pose of a Cow	Releasing tension in neck and shoulders
	The Mountain Pose	Relieve pressure from shoulders
Insomnia	Pose of a Cat Pose of a Locust	Relieve tension in spine and calming effects movements
	Slow Motion Firming	To calm the mind
	Complete Breath	To calm the mind

Premenstrual tension	Start each day with a 15-minute Miracle, except during period	To relieve tension
	Locust Positions	To relieve tension
Repetitive Stress injury	Start each day with a 15-minute Miracle	To help keep the spine tension free
	The Mountain Pose The Chest Expansion Pose of a Cow	All free the neck and shoulders from the tension resulting from overuse of the arms

I do hope that I have helped you understand the value and benefits of yoga in your life. Keep practicing often and you will do more for your body, mind, health, and feelings of wellbeing than you ever thought possible.

With my love
Barbara Currie

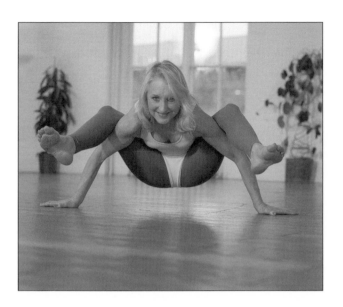

Using the Cards

The 30 cards give you three 15-minute yoga sequences, each one including the essentials such as breathing, stretching, relaxing, and balancing. Each of these 15-minute miracles will give you a perfectly balanced workout for mind and body. I would like you to start every day with one of these sequences. You'll be amazed at how quickly you will notice the difference. You will wonder how you ever began the day without them. They will keep your spine and joints really strong and flexible while toning virtually every muscle in your body. The sequences include magical toning exercises for the thighs and bottoms – great for smoothing out cellulite; abdominal exercises for really toning and firming the abdominals and slimming the midriff and the waistline; upper body exercises that tone and firm the arms and the muscles that support the bust; and those that concentrate on correcting posture, getting rid of tension in the neck and shoulders, and realigning the spine arms, necks, and bust.

Sequence one – Morning Essential

Have you ever watched an animal wake up after a rest? It stretches its body from top to toe. This gets rid of tension and makes sure it is in perfect condition to start the day. The first 15-minute miracle, Morning Essential, is an ideal sequence to start your day. It will greatly improve your shape and flexibility, give you bundles of

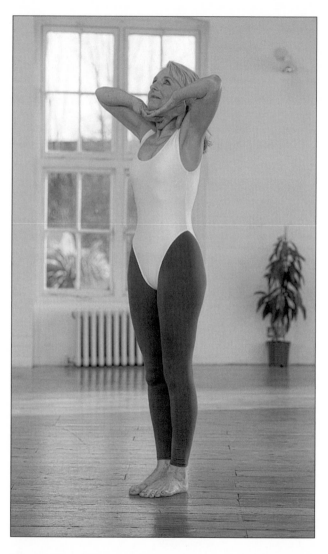

energy, and can be a tremendous help to people with an aching back. In my opinion, this simple 15-minute sequence is worth its weight in gold. It will give you energy, improve your shape, and is excellent for helping with and preventing back problems.

This first sequence – on cards 1 to 10 – is particularly suitable for beginners but those of you who are more experienced will know that in yoga the postures that seem to be the most simple can also be the strongest. Even when you feel as though you know a pose inside out, you will always find something more in it when you revisit it. That's the beauty of yoga, and it's also why yoga is a non-competitive system. Your flexibility will grow and grow – and in only 15 minutes a day!

Sequence two – the Advanced Miracle

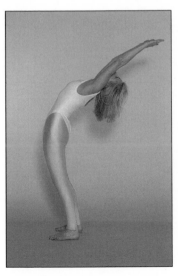

In the second 15-minute sequence you will move into more advanced yoga, that will stretch you a little more, in every sense of the word! In particular in the second sequence, the Advanced Miracle, there is the wonderful Salute to the Sun (see cards 12 and 13), the truly energizing morning stretch sequence practiced by many all over the world. This may take some time to

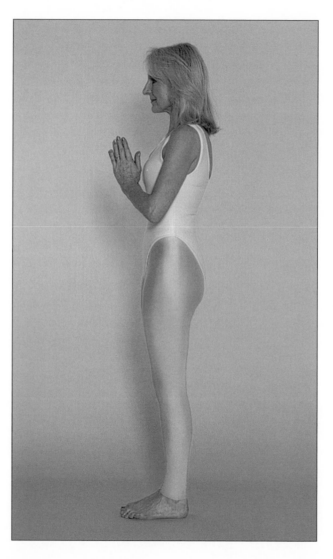

learn but practicing with the cards will help you remember and you will soon find yourself reaping the benefits of this wonderful exercise that in itself sets you up for the day.

Working on the breath is essential in yoga. In this second 15-minute sequence, the Advanced Miracle you will discover the wonder of the Complete Breath (see card 11), an exercise which teaches us to use the whole lung – for adequate oxygen absorption and higher energy levels. The two parts of the Pose of a Cat (see cards 16 and 17) give you the benefits of the kind of animal stretch that keeps a cat ready for action and free from tension. The second part of Pose of a Cat is really helpful for aching backs and it tones and firms the wrists, arms, thighs, and bottom. In the Advanced Miracle, the Big Toe Balance (see card 20), almost a sequence in itself, is wonderful for toning and firming the back of your thighs and for getting rid of cellulite.

As you will notice, there is also progression from the second to the third sequence. For instance, in the the Advanced Miracle you will learn the Half Locust pose (see card 15), which tones the bottom and thighs and releases tension in the lower back, followed by the Full Locust in the Third Wonder (see card 28), which greatly strengthens the lower back and helps to relieve constipation and menstrual troubles.

Sequence three – the Third Wonder

This third 15-minute sequence also shows you how to master the Warrior Sequence (see cards 23 and 24). As its name suggests, the Warrior Sequence is a posture of great strength. You will find it very empowering!

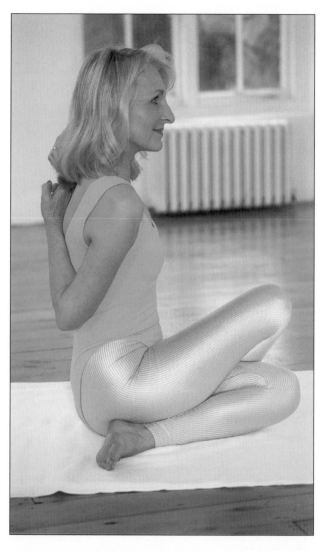

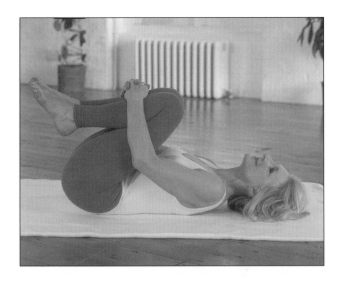

Yoga balances, another essential of yoga practice, tone, firm, and strengthen every muscle in the legs and bottom. They also teach us the power of concentration and focus and help to clear and concentrate the mind. There is a very special balance in the Third Wonder sequence: the Dancer's Posture is one of yoga's most beautiful movements (see card 25). As well as helping your concentration and balance, it will relieve tension in your lower back, and lift and firm your bottom. The Dancer's Posture also tones your thighs while strengthening the supporting leg.

The last card in the whole set of 30 is an absolute jewel. The Alternate Nostril Breathing Exercise (see card 30) is a very special part of yoga practice. It is calming and soothing and it will help you stay peaceful during difficult situations. It is particularly helpful to those suffering from congested sinuses. Alternate Nostril Breathing is ideal to do at night before you go to sleep but finding a couple of minutes to devote to your breath in a stressful day will pay dividends.

The cards give you a step-by-step instruction into sets of movements which will exercise and stretch you, relax you, and invigorate you. Enjoy!